ANTI-CANCER SURVIVAL GUIDE FOR SENIORS

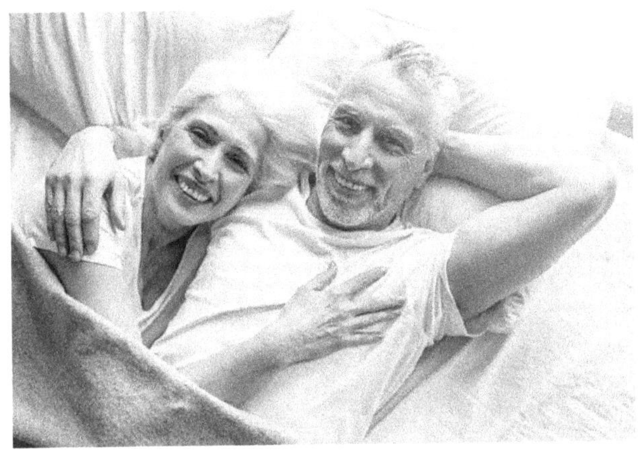

Comprehensive Guide for Surviving Cancer

Smart Desty

ANTI-CANCER SURVIVAL GUIDE FOR SENIORS

Table of Contents

ANTI-CANCER SURVIVAL GUIDE FOR SENIORS

INTRODUCTION

Cancer is one of the most common diseases among the elderly, with more than one in three seniors having been diagnosed with the disease. It can be a difficult and challenging journey for seniors and their families, and it's important to know the available resources and options for dealing with the illness. An "anti-cancer survival guide for seniors" is a valuable resource to help seniors and their families better understand the diagnosis, treatment options, and support services that are available.

A good anti-cancer survival guide for seniors should begin with a discussion of the basics of cancer, including the different types, how they are diagnosed, and the available treatment options. It should also provide information on the resources available to help seniors and their families cope with the diagnosis and treatment. This includes support groups, financial assistance, and educational resources.

Once the basics of cancer have been established, the anti-cancer survival guide should provide seniors with a comprehensive overview of the various treatments available. This should include information on chemotherapy, radiation, and surgery, as well as alternative treatments such as immunotherapy and natural therapies.

In addition to the information on treatments, the anti-cancer survival guide should also provide seniors with information on how to handle the emotional and spiritual aspects of their cancer journey. This includes tips on how to cope with stress, anxiety, and depression, as well as resources for finding psychological and spiritual support. The guide should also provide information on how to create a supportive environment for seniors and their families, such as joining a support group or finding a local cancer support center.

An important part of the anti-cancer survival guide for seniors should also be a discussion of preventive care and early detection. As the risk of cancer increases with age, it is important for seniors to take steps to reduce their risk. This includes avoiding exposure to carcinogens, eating a healthy diet, maintaining a healthy weight, and avoiding tobacco products. Additionally, seniors should receive regular checkups and screenings, such as mammograms, colonoscopies, and prostate exams, to detect cancer early. Early detection and diagnosis is key to successful cancer treatment, and this should be emphasized in the guide.

It is also important for the anti-cancer survival guide to provide seniors with information on how to access medical care. This includes information on the different types of health insurance available, as well as information on how to find a doctor, hospital, or other medical facility. Additionally, the guide should provide information on how to find a cancer specialist and how to access specialized care for particular types of cancer.

The anti-cancer survival guide should provide seniors with information on how to stay connected with their loved ones and support network during their cancer journey.

By providing seniors with a comprehensive overview of the diagnosis, treatment options, resources, and support services available, an anti-cancer survival guide can be a valuable resource for seniors and their families. With the right information and support, seniors can make informed decisions about their care and treatment and navigate their cancer journey with confidence.

ANTI-CANCER SURVIVAL GUIDE FOR SENIORS

Chapter One:
Understanding Cancer in Seniors

Cancer is a diagnosis that no one wants to hear, but it is a reality for many seniors. As the population of seniors grows, so too does the number of cancer diagnoses. Understanding cancer in seniors is important to ensure they receive the best possible care and treatment.

Cancer is a disease in which abnormal cells divide and spread uncontrollably. It results from changes in the DNA of a cell and can affect any tissue or organ in the body. Although cancer is most commonly found in adults, it can also occur in children and seniors.

Seniors are more likely to have cancer than younger adults due to their age. As people age, their cells become more susceptible to DNA damage, which can lead to cancer. Additionally, seniors are more likely to have built up a lifetime of exposure to environmental factors such as tobacco smoke, radiation, and certain chemicals, which can increase the risk of developing cancer.

Seniors can be diagnosed with any type of cancer, but some cancers are more common in this age group. The most common types of cancer in seniors are breast cancer, prostate cancer, lung cancer, and colorectal cancer. Other types of cancer such as skin cancer and leukemia can also occur in older adults.

It is important to note that the signs and symptoms of cancer in seniors may be different than those in younger adults. Seniors may experience fatigue, weight loss, and changes in appetite. They may also have difficulty sleeping, pain, and changes in bowel habits.

It is important for seniors to have regular check-ups and screenings to identify any potential health problems, including cancer. Early detection of cancer can increase the chances of successful treatment. After diagnosis, seniors should discuss all treatment options with their doctor.

Treatment options for cancer in seniors can include surgery, chemotherapy, radiation, and targeted therapy. The type of treatment and its effectiveness depend on the type of cancer, the stage of the cancer, and the overall health of the senior.

The side effects of cancer treatment can be more severe in seniors. Common side effects of chemotherapy can include fatigue, nausea, hair loss, and anemia. Radiation therapy can cause skin irritation, fatigue, and nausea. It is important for seniors to discuss their treatment options with their doctor to determine which is best for them.

Cancer in seniors can be a difficult and emotional process. It is important for seniors to have support from family, friends, and health care providers. It is also important to make sure that seniors have access to the best possible care, including support services such as counseling and physical therapy.

Understanding cancer in seniors is essential in order to ensure they receive the best possible care and treatment. Early detection and treatment can increase the chances of successful outcomes. It is important for seniors to have regular check-ups and screenings to identify any potential health problems, including cancer. Seniors should also discuss all treatment options with their doctor and have access to the best possible care.

It is also important for seniors to pay close attention to their own health and watch for any changes in their bodies. This includes keeping track of any changes in weight or appetite, as well as any new or worsening symptoms. Additionally, seniors should be sure to get enough sleep and exercise regularly.

Altering one's lifestyle can also lower a senior's risk of developing cancer. This includes quitting smoking, limiting alcohol consumption, and eating a healthy diet. It is also important to protect the skin from the sun and to avoid using tanning beds.

There is no one-size-fits-all approach to understanding cancer in seniors, but it is important to remember that early detection and treatment can increase the chances of successful outcomes. It is also important for seniors to have access to the best possible care and support services. By understanding cancer in seniors, we can help ensure that they receive the best possible care and treatment.

Chapter Two:

Preventing Cancer in Seniors

Cancer is a deadly disease that can affect people of any age, gender, or race. Seniors, in particular, are at an increased risk of developing cancer due to their age. However, there are a few things that seniors can do to reduce their risk of cancer and maintain a healthy lifestyle.

The first step in preventing cancer in seniors is to maintain a healthy lifestyle. This include maintaining a healthy weight, exercising frequently, and abstaining from tobacco use and binge drinking. Eating a balanced diet that includes fruits and vegetables can help reduce the risk of cancer in seniors. Regular exercise can also help seniors maintain their weight, which is important in keeping cancer risk low. Additionally, avoiding smoking and excessive alcohol consumption can help reduce the risk of cancer.

In addition to maintaining a healthy lifestyle, seniors should also receive regular check-ups from their doctor. These check-ups can help detect any signs of cancer early on, which can increase the chances of successful treatment. During these check-ups, the doctor will conduct a physical exam and may also order blood tests or other tests to look for signs of cancer. Seniors should also discuss any family history of cancer with their doctor and ask about the types of screening tests that are recommended for their age.

Seniors should also be aware of their environment and the potential risks that are associated with it. Exposure to certain environmental toxins and pollutants can increase the risk of cancer in seniors. They should avoid contact with any substances that they suspect may be harmful and limit their exposure to sunlight to reduce the risk of skin cancer.

In addition to lifestyle changes and regular check-ups, seniors should also consider participating in clinical trials. Clinical trials are research projects that evaluate the safety and efficacy of novel therapies or techniques. Seniors may benefit from taking part in clinical trials because they may gain access to cutting-edge treatments or procedures that aren't yet commonly used.

It is important for seniors to talk to their doctor about their cancer risk and the best ways to reduce their risk. Doctors can provide valuable information about cancer prevention and the latest treatments available. They can also provide emotional support and help seniors create an individualized treatment plan that fits their needs and lifestyle.

Seniors should also be aware of any changes in their bodies and report any unusual symptoms to their doctor. Unexplained changes in weight, fatigue, or appetite can be signs of cancer and should be discussed with a doctor right away. Additionally, seniors should be mindful of any changes in their skin and report any new moles or lesions to their doctor.

Seniors should also stay up to date on the latest cancer screenings and treatments available. They should talk to their doctor about the types of screenings that are recommended for their age and schedule regular screenings as needed. Additionally, they should be aware of new treatments and therapies that are available and ask their doctor about any that may be beneficial for them.

Cancer prevention is an important part of maintaining health and well-being for seniors. There are many steps that seniors can take to reduce their risk of cancer, including maintaining a healthy lifestyle, receiving regular check-ups from the doctor, and staying informed about the latest treatments and screenings. Additionally, seniors should be aware of any environmental toxins and pollutants that may increase their risk of cancer and limit their exposure to them.

Finally, it is important for seniors to stay active and maintain a positive attitude.

By taking steps to reduce their risk of cancer, seniors can live a long and healthy life. It is important for seniors to speak with their doctor about their cancer risk and the best ways to reduce it. With the right steps and the right attitude, seniors can reduce their risk of cancer and live a life of health and vitality.

Chapter Three:

Cancer Screenings for Seniors

Cancer screenings for seniors are an important part of maintaining good health and preventing the development of cancer. Early detection of cancer can increase the chances of successful treatment and prevent the spread of the disease. However, many seniors may not be aware of the different types of screenings available and the benefits they offer.

The most common type of cancer screening for seniors is a Pap test. This test looks for abnormal cells in the cervix and is usually recommended for women over the age of 21. Pap tests are usually performed every three to five years, depending on the results of the previous test. It is important to follow the recommended guidelines for Pap testing and to discuss any changes or concerns with a doctor.

A mammogram is an additional cancer screening option for elders. This screening looks for abnormalities in the breast tissue and is typically recommended for women over the age of 40. Mammograms are usually performed every two years and may be done more often for those at higher risk of breast cancer.

Another screening test that is suggested for males over 50 is the prostate-specific antigen (PSA) test. This test looks for elevated levels of a protein produced by the prostate gland and is typically done every year. Abnormal results may indicate an increased risk of prostate cancer and further testing may be recommended.

Colon cancer screening is also important for seniors, especially those over the age of 50. This screening looks for precancerous growths in the colon and rectum and can help identify cancer in its earliest stages. The most common screening method is a colonoscopy, which is typically done every 10 years. There are also other tests available, such as fecal occult blood tests and sigmoidoscopies, which may be recommended for those at higher risk of colon cancer.

Skin cancer screenings are important for seniors as well. During a skin cancer screening, a doctor will look for any signs of skin cancer, such as abnormal moles or discolored patches.

It is important to see a doctor if any changes or unusual spots are noticed.

Although cancer screenings are important for seniors, it is important to keep in mind that these tests can have risks and side effects. For example, the Pap test and mammograms can be uncomfortable and may cause some discomfort. Additionally, a colonoscopy or biopsy may be necessary if cancer is suspected and these tests can have more serious side effects. It is important to discuss the risks and benefits of each screening test with a doctor before making a decision.

It is essential for seniors to be aware that cancer screenings are not foolproof. While these tests can help detect cancer in its early stages, they cannot always detect all forms of cancer. It is important to be aware of any symptoms of cancer and to see a doctor if there are any changes or concerns.

Overall, cancer screenings are an important part of maintaining good health for seniors. Early detection of cancer can increase the chances of successful treatment and prevent the spread of the disease. It is important to discuss the risks and benefits of each screening test with a doctor before making a decision and to be aware of any symptoms of cancer.

Cancer screenings for seniors are an important tool in preventing the development of cancer and monitoring existing diseases. Screening tests such as Pap tests, mammograms, PSA tests, colonoscopies, and skin cancer screenings can help detect cancer in its early stages and provide a greater chance of successful treatment. Seniors should discuss the risks and benefits of each test with their doctor and be aware of any symptoms of cancer.

In addition to the cancer screenings mentioned above, there are also other tests available for seniors. For example, a physical exam can help detect any changes in the body that may be indicative of cancer. Additionally, blood tests may be recommended to detect certain types of cancer, such as ovarian and prostate cancer. Finally, imaging tests, such as X-rays, CT scans, and MRIs, may be used to detect cancer in various organs.

It is important for seniors to understand the importance of regular cancer screenings and to work with their doctor to determine which tests are necessary and how often they should be done. Screenings can be uncomfortable and may have risks and side effects, so it is important to discuss these with a doctor before making a decision. Additionally, it is important to be aware that cancer screenings are not foolproof and may not detect all forms of cancer.

Cancer screenings are an important way for seniors to maintain good health and reduce the risk of developing cancer. It is important to discuss the risks and benefits of each test with a doctor and to be aware of any symptoms of cancer. Early detection can increase the chances of successful treatment, so it is important for seniors to get regular screenings and to follow their doctor's advice.

Chapter Four:

Understanding Cancer Treatments

Cancer treatments are an ever-evolving field of medical science. With advances in technology and medical knowledge, treatments are becoming more effective and less invasive. Understanding the different treatments available to patients is key in making informed decisions about their health care.

Treatment for cancer is determined by the type of cancer, its stage, and overall health of the patient. Surgery, chemotherapy, radiation, and immunotherapy are the most commonly used cancer treatments.

Surgery is the oldest and most commonly used treatment for cancer. Depending on the type and stage of cancer, surgery may be used to remove the tumor and surrounding tissue, or to perform biopsies to determine the extent of the disease. Surgery can also be used to prepare a patient for other treatments, such as radiation or chemotherapy.

Chemotherapy is the use of drugs to kill cancer cells. Drugs are typically given intravenously or orally, depending on the type of cancer. Chemotherapy is effective at killing cancer cells, but can also damage healthy cells. Side effects can include fatigue, hair loss, nausea, and infection. Some newer forms of chemotherapy are targeted, meaning they are designed to attack specific cancer cells while leaving healthy cells intact.

Radiation therapy is the use of high-energy beams of radiation to kill cancer cells. External beam radiation is the most common type of radiation therapy, and involves directing radiation from a machine outside the body to the affected area. This type of therapy is used to shrink tumors or kill any remaining cancer cells after surgery. Internal radiation, or brachytherapy, involves placing radioactive material directly into the tumor or affected area.

Immunotherapy is a type of treatment that uses the body's own immune system to fight cancer. Immunotherapy encourages the immune system to identify and fight cancer cells. This type of treatment is often used when other cancer treatments have been unsuccessful, or when the cancer has spread to other parts of the body.

Most cancer treatments have side effects, and these can vary depending on the type and extent of treatment. Common side effects of chemotherapy and radiation include fatigue, hair loss, nausea, and infection. Surgery may also lead to side effects such as pain, swelling, and scarring.

In addition to the treatments listed above, there are also newer forms of cancer treatments that are being studied and developed. These include gene therapy, which involves using modified genes to target and kill cancer cells, and photodynamic therapy, which uses light-activated drugs to kill cancer cells.

The effectiveness of cancer treatments varies from person to person, and it is important to discuss all of the available options with a doctor before deciding on a treatment plan. Understanding the different types of treatments available, as well as the potential side effects, is key to making an informed decision about cancer treatment.

Complementary and alternative treatments for cancer can also be used in conjunction with traditional treatments. These treatments can include herbal medicines, dietary changes, acupuncture, massage therapy, and other lifestyle modifications. While there is limited evidence to support the effectiveness of these treatments, some studies suggest that they may improve quality of life and reduce symptoms.

It is important to note that emotional support and understanding from family and friends is essential in helping a person cope with a cancer diagnosis and treatment. Support groups can provide a safe space to discuss fears and concerns, as well as to connect with other individuals in similar situations. Additionally, talking with a counselor, psychologist, or social worker can help a person develop coping mechanisms, manage stress, and find emotional support.

Cancer treatments are constantly evolving and understanding the different treatments available is key in making informed decisions about health care. Surgery, chemotherapy, radiation, and immunotherapy are the most common forms of traditional treatments, while complementary and alternative treatments may also be used. Additionally, emotional support from family and friends, as well as from professionals, is essential in helping a person cope with the diagnosis and treatment of cancer. With the right tools, patients can make informed decisions, manage their symptoms, and lead a healthy life.

Chapter Five:

Choosing a Treatment Plan

Choosing a Treatment Plan is a crucial step for anyone who is suffering from a medical condition or a mental health issue. The decision is not always easy and it is important to consider all of the options available and to make an informed decision before proceeding.

When selecting a treatment plan, the first step is to review the diagnosis and to understand the cause of the condition or issue. This will help to determine what type of treatment is best suited to the individual. In addition to understanding the diagnosis, it is important to understand the different treatment options available and the benefits and risks associated with each.

It is important to talk to a healthcare provider or mental health professional and to discuss all of the available options. This is important in order to make sure that the right type of treatment is chosen. It is also important to find out what type of support is available to the patient during and after the treatment plan.

It is also important to take into consideration the cost of the treatment plan. Treatment plans can be expensive and can be difficult to afford. It is important to consider all of the options available and to determine which is the most cost-effective.

When choosing a treatment plan, it is also important to consider the patient's lifestyle. Some treatment plans may require the patient to make changes to their lifestyle or to make changes to their diet and exercise routine. It is important to understand what changes will be required and to make sure that the patient is willing and able to make these changes.

It is also important to take into consideration the patient's expectations for the treatment plan. It is important to understand what the patient expects from the treatment plan and to make sure that these expectations are realistic.

It is crucial to consider the long-term effects of the treatment plan. It is important to understand how the treatment plan will affect the patient's life in the long-term and to make sure that the patient is comfortable with the long-term effects.

Choosing a treatment plan is a difficult decision, but it is an important one. It is important to consider all of the options available and to make an informed decision. It is also important to talk to a healthcare provider or mental health professional and to discuss all of the available options. Finally, it is important to consider the cost of the treatment plan, the patient's lifestyle, their expectations, and the long-term effects. Taking all of these factors into consideration can help to ensure that the best treatment plan is chosen.

Chapter Six:

Understanding Cancer Prognosis

Cancer prognosis is an assessment of the likely course of a cancer in terms of the response to treatment, length of survival, and the quality of life. It is an essential component of cancer management as it helps to guide treatment decisions and to plan supportive care for the patient. The prognosis is based on the type of cancer, its stage, the individual's age, and other factors such as the patient's overall health and the treatment they receive.

Cancer prognosis is based on the specific characteristics of each individual patient's cancer. As such, no two prognoses are exactly the same. A cancer prognosis is more of a prediction than a certainty. It is an estimate of the outcome of a patient's cancer based on the information available at the time of assessment. The prognosis can change over time as new information becomes available or if the cancer progresses or responds to treatment.

When assessing a patient's prognosis, the doctor will consider several factors, including the type and stage of the cancer, the person's age and overall health, the location of the primary tumor, and the extent of spread of the cancer. Other factors that may be taken into account include the patient's lifestyle, available treatments, and the patient's response to treatment.

Cancer prognosis is expressed in terms of the cancer's expected duration or survival rate. Survival rates are based on the number of people with a certain type of cancer who are still alive a certain number of years after being diagnosed. The rate may be expressed as a percentage or as a median survival time. For example, a 5-year survival rate of 90 percent means that 90 percent of the people with the cancer are still alive five years after diagnosis. The median survival time means that half of the people with the cancer are still alive at the stated number of years after diagnosis.

The prognosis of a person with cancer can also be expressed in terms of the expected quality of life. Quality of life is affected by many factors, including the patient's response to treatment, the side effects of treatment, the level of pain and other symptoms, and the emotional impact of the diagnosis and treatment.

Cancer prognosis is important in helping the patient and their family understand the likely course of the disease and the options available for treatment and support. It can also be used to plan for the future, such as making arrangements for life after treatment or making decisions about end-of-life care.

Cancer prognosis is a complex and difficult process. It is important that the doctor and patient discuss the prognosis in detail and that any questions or concerns the patient may have are addressed. It is also important that the patient be given support and information to help them cope with the diagnosis and treatment.

Chapter Seven:

Coping with a Cancer Diagnosis

Coping with a cancer diagnosis can be an incredibly difficult challenge to face. It can be a source of fear, stress, and other strong emotions. It's important to understand that it is normal to feel this way and to recognize the need for support. It is also important to remember that everyone's experience is unique and there is no one "right" way to cope with a cancer diagnosis.

The first step in coping with a cancer diagnosis is to accept it. It is important to acknowledge the reality of the situation and to recognize that it will not go away on its own. Once the diagnosis is accepted, it is important to learn as much as possible about the cancer, including what type it is, what treatments may be available, and what the prognosis is. It can also be helpful to talk to a medical professional and to join a support group to connect with others who are going through a similar experience.

It is also important to take care of oneself while coping with a cancer diagnosis. This includes getting enough rest, eating healthy foods, and exercising regularly. It is also important to find healthy ways to cope with emotions such as fear, anger, and sadness. This could include talking to a friend, writing in a journal, or engaging in activities that bring joy.

In addition to the practicalities of coping with a cancer diagnosis, it is important to remember to take time to appreciate the good things in life. This could include spending time with family and friends, engaging in activities that bring pleasure and relaxation, and practicing mindfulness or meditation.

It is important to recognize that no one should have to cope with a cancer diagnosis alone. Family and friends can be a great source of support during this time. It is also important to find a support group that can provide emotional support and understanding.

Cancer can be a difficult and frightening experience, and it is important to remember that everyone copes differently. Taking the time to acknowledge the reality of the situation, to learn as much as possible about the cancer and its treatment, and to take care of oneself while engaging in activities that bring joy and relaxation can all be beneficial. Additionally, it is important to remember that no one should have to cope with a cancer diagnosis alone, and that there are resources and support systems available to help.

It is also crucial to remember that everyone's cancer journey is unique, and that there is no "right" way to cope with a cancer diagnosis. Everyone's experience and needs are different, and it is important to find what works best for oneself. It is also important to recognize that it is normal to have a wide range of emotions, including fear, anger, and sadness, and to find healthy ways to express and manage these emotions.

In addition to seeking emotional support, it can also be beneficial to engage in activities that promote physical and mental health. This could include getting enough rest, eating healthy foods, and exercising regularly. It can also be beneficial to practice mindfulness or meditation and to engage in activities that bring joy and relaxation. This could include spending time with family and friends, going for walks in nature, listening to music, or engaging in hobbies that bring pleasure.

It is also important to remember that there are resources available to help those coping with a cancer diagnosis. Organizations such as the American Cancer Society can provide information and support. Additionally, talking to a medical professional or joining a support group can be helpful.

It is important to remember to keep hope alive. Everyone's cancer journey is unique, and it is important to recognize that there is always a chance that things will get better. It is also important to remember that no one should have to cope with a cancer diagnosis alone, and to seek support when needed.

Chapter Eight:

Finding Support During Cancer Treatment

Cancer treatment can be a difficult and draining experience. It can be an emotionally and physically grueling journey that can take a toll on the spirit, mind, and body. The process can be overwhelming, and many people facing cancer treatment feel isolated, alone, and in need of support. Finding support during cancer treatment is essential for maintaining physical and emotional health.

When going through cancer treatment, it is important to build a support system. Family and friends can provide much-needed support, as well as practical and emotional assistance. They can offer a listening ear and provide encouragement to those undergoing cancer treatment. It is also helpful to join a support group, either in person or online. These support groups provide a safe, non-judgmental space to share experiences and connect with others who are facing similar challenges.

It is also important to look for professional help, such as a counselor or therapist. A counselor or therapist can provide emotional support, help you cope with the stress of cancer treatment, and develop strategies to manage difficult feelings and emotions. A counselor or therapist can also provide support for family members who are affected by the cancer diagnosis.

Complementary therapies can also be helpful for providing support during cancer treatment. These therapies are not intended to replace conventional treatments. Instead, they can be used to provide additional support to help reduce stress, manage pain, and improve quality of life. Examples of complementary therapies include acupuncture, massage, yoga, meditation, and relaxation techniques.

Many people find that spiritual support is helpful during cancer treatment. Churches, synagogues, and other religious organizations can provide spiritual guidance and support. Spending time in nature can also be helpful, as nature can provide healing, solace, and a sense of peace.

It's crucial to keep in mind that everyone has distinct demands. Some people may find that talking to a close friend or family member is helpful, while others may need to join a support group or talk to a professional. The most important thing is to find what works for you and to find the support that you need.

Cancer treatment can be a difficult and overwhelming process, but it is important to remember that you are not alone. There are many resources available to provide support during cancer treatment. From family and friends to support groups and professional help, there are many ways to find the support you need. It is important to take the time to find the resources that can help you through this challenging time.

It is also important to stay connected with your healthcare team during cancer treatment. Your healthcare team can provide valuable information, answer questions, and suggest resources that can provide additional support. Additionally, they can provide advice and support on how to manage the side effects of cancer treatment and provide resources for additional support.

Be very diligent to take care of yourself during cancer treatment. Ensure that you get adequate sleep, exercise, and consume a balanced diet. Exercise can help reduce stress and improve energy levels. Additionally, connecting with friends and family members can help reduce stress and provide emotional support.

Always remember that cancer treatment is a journey and it is important to take time to process the emotions that come with it. Taking time for yourself and doing activities that you enjoy can help to reduce stress, provide a sense of normalcy, and provide a sense of control.

Finding support during cancer treatment is essential for managing the physical and emotional challenges of the journey. It is important to build a support system and find the resources that are right for you. Whether it is family and friends, a support group, a counselor or therapist, complementary therapies, or spiritual support, finding the support you need during cancer treatment can help you to cope with the challenges, manage stress, and maintain physical and emotional health.

Chapter Nine:

Managing Side Effects of Cancer Treatment

Managing the side effects of cancer treatment is an important part of the recovery process. Cancer treatment can cause a range of physical and emotional side effects, and it is important to take steps to manage these side effects in order to maintain a good quality of life during treatment and recovery. This can include a variety of strategies, such as eating a healthy diet, getting enough rest, exercising regularly, using stress-relieving techniques, and talking to a doctor or other healthcare professional about any medication side effects.

The most common side effects of cancer treatment are fatigue, nausea, vomiting, hair loss, and changes in taste. These side effects can vary in severity and duration, and they can affect different people in different ways. It is important to talk to a doctor or healthcare professional about any side effects that are experienced and to ask for advice on how to manage them.

Eating a healthy diet can help to reduce some of the side effects of cancer treatment. Eating a diet high in fruits and vegetables, whole grains, and lean proteins can help to provide the body with the energy and nutrients it needs to stay healthy and cope with the side effects of treatment. It is also important to drink plenty of fluids and to get enough rest.

Exercising regularly can also help to reduce some of the side effects of cancer treatment. Exercise can help to reduce fatigue, improve mood, and maintain muscle strength. It can also help to reduce nausea and vomiting. It is important to talk to a doctor or healthcare professional before starting a new exercise routine, and to start slowly and gradually increase the intensity.

Managing stress is also an important part of managing side effects of cancer treatment. Stress can worsen side effects and make them more difficult to manage. Stress-relieving techniques such as meditation, yoga, and deep breathing can help to reduce stress and improve overall wellbeing. It is also important to try to maintain a positive outlook and to make time for enjoyable activities.

Medication can also be used to manage the side effects of cancer treatment. Some medications can help to reduce nausea and vomiting, while others can help to reduce fatigue or improve mood. It is important to talk to a doctor or healthcare professional about any medication side effects and to ask for advice on how to manage them.

Managing the side effects of cancer treatment can be challenging, but there are a variety of strategies that can be used to help manage them. Eating a healthy diet, getting enough rest, exercising regularly, and managing stress can help to reduce some of the side effects. Medication can also be used to manage side effects, and it is important to talk to a doctor or healthcare professional about any medication side effects and to ask for advice on how to manage them. Taking steps to manage side effects can help to improve quality of life during treatment and recovery.

It can also be helpful to talk to other people who are going through cancer treatment, or who have been through it. They may be able to provide advice, support, and understanding. It can also be helpful to take time out for yourself and to do activities that you enjoy. This can help to reduce stress, improve mood, and provide a sense of normalcy during a difficult time.

It is important to be aware of the signs and symptoms of cancer treatment side effects and to seek medical help if needed. Common signs of cancer treatment side effects include pain, fatigue, nausea, vomiting, and changes in appetite. If any of these side effects become severe or persist for more than a few days, it is important to seek medical help.

Managing the side effects of cancer treatment can be challenging, but there are a variety of strategies that can be used to help manage them. Taking steps to eat a healthy diet, get enough rest, exercise regularly, manage stress, and talk to a doctor or healthcare professional about any medication side effects can help to reduce some of the side effects and improve overall quality of life during treatment and recovery.

Chapter Ten:

Practical Considerations During Treatment

Practical considerations during treatment refer to the various strategies and guidelines that therapists and clients should adhere to in order to ensure an effective and successful therapy session. These considerations are vital to the success of a therapy session, as they help to create an environment that is conducive to productive and meaningful conversations. Practical considerations during treatment can also help to ensure that the therapist and client are comfortable and that the therapy session runs smoothly and efficiently.

The first practical consideration during treatment is to ensure that there is a safe and comfortable environment. This means that the therapist should create an atmosphere that is conducive to open and honest communication between the therapist and client. This includes ensuring that the space is free from distraction and noise, is private, and is comfortable for both the therapist and the client. It is also important that the therapist and client feel comfortable with one another and that they are both willing to participate in the therapy session.

The second practical consideration during treatment is to ensure that the therapist and client are both prepared for the session. This means that the therapist should have a clear understanding of the client's goals and objectives for the session and that the therapist is prepared to help the client work towards these goals. It is also important that the therapist and client both have a clear understanding of the therapy process and that they both have an understanding of the techniques that the therapist plans to use during the session.

The third practical consideration during treatment is to ensure that the therapist and client agree on the goals and objectives of the session. It is important that the therapist and client both have an understanding of the goals and objectives that they are working towards and that they both agree on how these goals and objectives will be accomplished. This includes agreeing on the frequency of sessions, the length of the sessions, and other specific details of the therapy process.

The fourth practical consideration during treatment is to ensure that the therapist and client have a clear understanding of the progress the client has made and the progress that still needs to be made. This means that the therapist should regularly assess the progress that the client has made and that the therapist should make sure that the client is still making progress towards the goals and objectives that have been set. This assessment should include an assessment of the progress that has been made in terms of the client's mental health and emotional well-being, as well as in terms of the progress that has been made in terms of the client's goals and objectives.

The fifth practical consideration during treatment is to ensure that the therapist and client are both aware of any challenges or obstacles that the client is facing. This means that the therapist should be aware of any potential triggers or stressors that the client may be facing and that the therapist should be prepared to help the client address these challenges. This includes understanding the client's coping strategies and helping the client to develop new coping strategies that are effective for managing the challenges and stressors that the client is facing.

The sixth practical consideration during treatment is to ensure that the therapist and client both understand the importance of confidentiality. This means that the therapist should ensure that the client's privacy and confidentiality are respected and that the client's information is kept confidential. This includes understanding the laws and regulations that govern the client's privacy and confidentiality and making sure that the client's information is not shared with anyone without the client's permission.

The seventh practical consideration during treatment is to ensure that the therapist and client both understand the importance of feedback and communication. This means that the therapist should regularly provide feedback to the client about the progress that the client has made and the progress that still needs to be made. This feedback should be provided in an honest and open manner and should be tailored to the individual needs of the client. Additionally, the therapist should ensure that the client feels comfortable providing feedback to the therapist and that the therapist is open to receiving feedback from the client.

Finally, the eighth practical consideration during treatment is to ensure that the therapist and client both understand the importance of follow-up. This means that the therapist should ensure that the client is regularly seen by the therapist after the therapy session is complete and that the therapist is available to answer any questions or concerns that the client may have. Additionally, the therapist should ensure that the client is provided with resources and support that can help the client continue to make progress towards their goals and objectives.

By adhering to the practical considerations during treatment, therapists and clients can ensure that the therapy session is productive and meaningful and that the therapy process is successful. Practical considerations during treatment can help to create an environment that is conducive to open and honest communication between the therapist and client and can help to ensure that the therapist and client are both comfortable and prepared for the therapy session. Additionally, these considerations can help to ensure that the client is making progress towards the goals and objectives set for the session and that the client is receiving the necessary resources and support to continue to make progress.

Chapter Eleven:

Integrative and Complementary Therapies

Integrative and complementary therapies are treatments used in addition to traditional medicine to help treat and manage health conditions. These therapies may include physical, psychological and spiritual approaches. They are often used to supplement traditional medical treatments to provide additional relief from symptoms, as well as to promote overall health and wellbeing.

Integrative and complementary therapies are used in a variety of settings, including hospitals, clinics, and in the home. They can be used to treat a wide range of health conditions, from physical ailments such as chronic pain to psychological issues like depression and anxiety. They can also be used to help with lifestyle changes, such as quitting smoking or managing stress.

The goal of integrative and complementary therapies is to provide relief from symptoms while also taking into account the patient's individual needs and preferences. These therapies often focus on the whole person, including their physical, emotional, mental, and spiritual health. They may include mindfulness-based practices, such as meditation and yoga, as well as more traditional methods like acupuncture and massage.

Integrative and complementary therapies are often used in conjunction with traditional medical treatments. For example, a patient may be prescribed medication for a medical condition, but may also benefit from massage therapy or acupuncture to help manage their symptoms. This approach is known as integrative medicine, and it seeks to combine the best of traditional and alternative medicine.

The use of integrative and complementary therapies is increasing, and it is becoming more accepted by the medical community. In some cases, these therapies are even covered by health insurance. However, it is important to note that these therapies are not a substitute for traditional medical treatment. It is important to discuss any integrative or complementary therapies with your doctor before beginning any treatments.

Integrative and complementary therapies can be used to promote overall health and wellbeing, as well as to manage specific health conditions. It is important to remember that these therapies are used to supplement traditional medical treatments, and should not be used as a substitute. It is also important to discuss any therapies with your doctor before beginning any treatments, as some therapies may interact with traditional medications.

The utilization of integrative and complementary therapies is becoming more widespread, and more research is being done to assess their effectiveness and safety. While these therapies can provide relief from symptoms and promote overall health and wellbeing, it is important to remember that they should be used in conjunction with traditional medical treatments. This approach can help individuals achieve their desired health outcomes and experience improved quality of life.

79

Chapter Twelve:

Nutrition and Cancer

Nutrition and cancer are two topics that are closely related. Nutrition is essential for providing the energy and nutrients that are needed to maintain healthy cells, while cancer is a disease caused by abnormal cell growth. Eating a healthy and balanced diet is one of the most important steps that people can take to reduce the risk of developing cancer. There are many ways that nutrition can affect cancer, including providing the body with essential nutrients, reducing inflammation, and helping to maintain a healthy body weight.

Good nutrition is essential for preventing and managing cancer. Eating a healthy and balanced diet can provide the body with the nutrients it needs to fight off cancer cells, while also helping to reduce the risk of developing cancer in the future. Eating plenty of fruits and vegetables, whole grains, and lean proteins can help to provide the body with the essential vitamins and minerals it needs to stay healthy. Additionally, limiting processed foods, refined sugars, and saturated fats can help to reduce the risk of developing cancer.

In addition to providing essential nutrients, eating a healthy diet can also help to reduce inflammation, which is a key factor in the development of cancer. Eating a diet rich in anti-inflammatory foods such as omega-3 fatty acids, monounsaturated fats, and antioxidants can help to reduce inflammation in the body, which can help to reduce the risk of developing cancer. Additionally, eating a diet low in animal fats and processed foods can help to reduce inflammation in the body.

Maintaining a healthy body weight is also essential for reducing the risk of developing cancer. Eating a healthy and balanced diet, as well as exercising regularly, can help to keep the body at a healthy weight. Being overweight or obese increases the risk of developing certain types of cancer, such as breast and colon cancer.

Finally, nutrition can also help to manage cancer once it has been diagnosed. Eating a healthy and balanced diet can help to provide the body with the energy and nutrients it needs to fight off cancer cells. Additionally, certain foods may be recommended depending on the type of cancer and the treatment plan. For example, a person with breast cancer may be advised to increase their intake of cruciferous vegetables, while a person with prostate cancer may be advised to increase their intake of soy products.

Nutrition plays an important role in both preventing and managing cancer. Eating a healthy and balanced diet can help to provide the body with the essential vitamins and minerals it needs to stay healthy, while also helping to reduce inflammation and maintain a healthy body weight. Additionally

Chapter Thirteen:

Exercise During Cancer

Exercise during cancer is an essential component of a healthy lifestyle. Cancer patients should be encouraged to maintain an active lifestyle, even if they cannot engage in vigorous activity. Research has shown that exercise can reduce fatigue, improve quality of life, reduce stress and anxiety, and even improve survival rates. Exercise can also help cancer patients manage the side effects of their treatment and improve their physical and emotional well-being.

Exercise can help cancer patients in a number of ways. First, it can help reduce fatigue. Cancer treatment frequently causes fatigue, which can make it difficult for a patient to stay active and engage in daily activities. Engaging in regular physical activity can help reduce fatigue and improve quality of life. Exercise can also help reduce stress and anxiety. Stress and anxiety can be caused by the physical and emotional changes associated with a cancer diagnosis. Exercise can help reduce stress and anxiety by providing an outlet for those feelings and improving mood.

Exercise has also been shown to improve survival rates in some cancer patients. Several studies have found that regular physical activity can reduce the risk of death from cancer. One study found that people who engaged in regular physical activity had a 16 percent lower risk of death from all causes, including cancer. Another study found that men with prostate cancer who engaged in regular physical activity had a 33 percent lower risk of death from the disease.

Exercise can also help cancer patients manage the side effects of their treatment. Chemotherapy and radiation can cause nausea, fatigue, and other unpleasant side effects. Exercise can help reduce these side effects by improving circulation, increasing energy levels, and reducing stress. Exercise can also help with pain management. Pain is a common side effect of cancer treatment, and exercise can help reduce pain by strengthening muscles and improving flexibility.

Exercise can help improve a person's emotional well-being. Cancer can be a difficult and emotional time, and exercise can provide a healthy outlet for stress and anxiety. Exercise can also help improve mood and self-esteem by helping individuals feel better about themselves and their situation.

Exercise during cancer can be beneficial for patients both physically and emotionally. However, it is important to consult with a doctor before starting any physical activity. Cancer patients should also be aware of their physical limitations and not push themselves too hard. Exercise should be tailored to each individual's needs, and patients should listen to their bodies and stop if they experience any pain or discomfort. With the right approach, exercise during cancer can help improve quality of life and even improve survival rates.

Chapter Fourteen:

Living with Cancer

It can be challenging to have cancer. It may tire you physically, mentally, and emotionally. It can be a long, hard journey with no easy answers. Living with cancer means learning to cope with the physical effects of the illness as well as dealing with the emotional and psychological issues that come along with it.

Firstly, a person living with cancer will have to learn to cope with the physical effects of the illness. This can include fatigue, pain, nausea, and other side effects of treatment. These effects can make it difficult to stay active and make it hard to keep up with day to day activities. It is important to get enough rest, stay hydrated, and eat healthy. Some people may also want to look into alternative treatments such as massage and acupuncture to help with pain management.

Secondly, living with cancer means dealing with the emotional and psychological issues that come along with it. This can include fear, depression, anxiety, and guilt. It is important to find a way to manage these emotions and find ways to cope. This could include talking to a therapist, joining a support group, or writing in a journal. It is also important to remember that emotions will fluctuate and it is okay to feel a range of emotions.

Thirdly, it is important to take care of oneself while living with cancer. This includes getting enough rest, eating nutritious foods, and exercising. It is also important to find ways to relax such as yoga, meditation, and spending time with family and friends. These activities help to reduce stress and can help maintain one's physical and mental wellbeing.

Fourthly, it is important to reach out to family and friends for support. It is important to talk to someone about how you are feeling and to seek help if needed. It is also important to remember that you are not alone in your journey and that there are people who are willing to help.

Finally, living with cancer means learning to accept the illness and finding ways to live a full and meaningful life. This may mean finding new ways to enjoy life and finding a new purpose. It can also mean learning to accept that life can be unpredictable and that it is okay to not have all the answers.

Living with cancer is not easy but it is possible. It is important to remember that it is a journey and that it is not something to be taken lightly. It is important to take care of yourself, reach out for help when needed, and find ways to live a full and meaningful life.

Conclusion

The Anti-cancer survival guide for seniors is a comprehensive guide to understanding and managing cancer. It is designed to empower seniors to make informed decisions about their cancer care and to provide them with resources to improve their quality of life. The guide covers topics such as prevention, diagnosis and treatment, as well as lifestyle changes that can help prevent cancer and improve overall health. It also includes tips on managing stress, managing finances, and getting the right support.

The guide provides seniors with the information they need to make informed decisions about their cancer care. The guide is comprehensive and covers a wide range of topics, from prevention and diagnosis to treatment and lifestyle changes. It also includes helpful information on managing stress, finances, and getting the right support.

The guide also provides seniors with resources to help them make the most of their cancer journey. These resources include support groups and organizations, financial assistance programs, and helpful websites. The guide also provides links to helpful websites and articles that can provide more information about cancer and how to best manage it.

The Anti-cancer survival guide for seniors is an invaluable resource for seniors living with cancer. It provides seniors with the tools and resources to make informed decisions about their cancer care, as well as tips and advice on managing their stress and finances and getting the right support. The guide is an invaluable resource for seniors who are facing a difficult and often scary journey. It provides them with the knowledge and resources to help make their cancer journey as successful and as stress-free as possible.